How To Survive
Snack Attacks
...Naturally

By Judi and Shari Zucker
"The Double-Energy Twins"

Foreword by
Paavo Airola, Ph.D., N.D.

Published by
Woodbridge Press Publishing Company
Santa Barbara, California 93111

Published by

Woodbridge Press Publishing Company
Post Office Box 6189
Sana Barbara, California 93111

Published simultaneously in the United States and Canada

Printed in the United States of America

Cover photos: Margo Vann Studio

Library of Congress Cataloging in Publication Data

Zucker, Judi.
   How to survive snack attacks . . . naturally.

   Includes index.
    1. Cookery (Natural foods) 2. Snack foods.
I. Zucker, Shari, joint author. II. Title.
TX741.Z82   641.8'1   79-12781
ISBN 0-912800-63-1

Dedication

We dedicate this book to our fantastic,
health-oriented, and fun-loving parents—Irwin and
Devra Hill Zucker—and to the many beautiful,
positive-thinking friends who kept asking for these
recipes for our "neat sweet treats."

Contents

A Foreword

Dr. Paavo Airola Says . . .
"Simply Delicious!"

It is refreshing to see a couple of youngsters becoming so involved in nutrition and healthful living that they write their first book. If this indicates the growing health and nutrition awareness among our young, then the future of the world may not be as dim as it sometimes seems.

Judi and Shari, the Zucker twins, fitness leaders and track stars at Beverly Hills High School, have put together a delightful collection of recipes for nutritious snacks—and these are their own recipes. I have sampled some of the end results—and they are simply delicious!

Although I am not an advocate of sweets, and although cookies, cakes, and desserts have no place in a strict Airola Optimum Diet, I recognize the importance of such "goodies" when there are younger people in the family. And since it is almost impossible to buy in stores high-quality snacks and desserts that would be totally natural, sugar-free, and without any harmful additives, this collection of natural snack recipes can fill an important gap in the growing library of recipe books.

Therefore, I am happy to recommend *How To Survive Snack Attacks—Naturally.*

Bon Appetit!

—*Paavo Airola, Ph.D., N.D.*

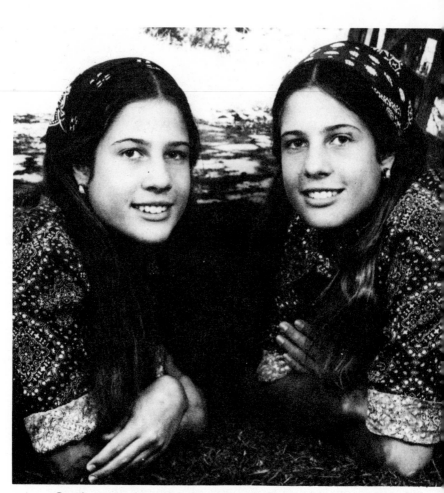

Good nutrition has to be taken seriously. That's why we have studied it so thoroughly. With good health you can have the fun that health makes possible.

Introduction

New and Creative Recipes

About four years ago, we became vegetarians and also decided to change our junk food eating habits. While exploring the world of health foods, to our disappointment we often found candies and pies made with sugar or preservatives. Even the sweets made out of honey were too sweet.

To satisfy our "snack attacks" and sweet-tooth cravings, we began to make up our own recipes. We studied nutrition and learned many new ideas. After experimenting with many foods, we developed new and creative recipes for cookies and pies. The more we cooked, the more we enjoyed our own foods.

How To Survive Snack Attacks—Naturally

The best thing about our goodies is that they aren't wasted calories. Very often, one will snack on potato chips or some refined white-floured and sugared-up cookies. These foods contain nothing but empty calories. In our recipes, we use only whole grains, whole eggs, and fresh fruit. We use no sugar, baking powder or soda, no artificial additives and no processed oils.

Also, don't worry about getting fat on our food. If you follow our advice about exercise and a balanced diet, you should have no trouble indulging yourself in these treats. They are also not highly concentrated or overdone. We try to minimize the oils and even natural sweeteners as much as possible without taking away from the flavor. We don't use salt, either. With all the other flavorings, it's not needed.

When a fruit isn't enough to satisfy your "snack attack," open up this book and bake. Remember, most of these snacks can be stored in the freezer and reheated whenever you want them.

We hope you enjoy these delicious and nutritious goodies as much as we do.

—"The Double-Energy Twins,"
Judi and Shari Zucker

List of Recipes and Topics

Recipes

To Your Taste!

If some of the recipes are not sweet enough for your personal taste, simply add any of the natural sweeteners (tupelo honey, fructose, maple syrup, or dried, crushed dates) to please your palate.

Double-Your-Energy Health Drink

. . . for pleasant sipping with the treats in this book . . . or for a quick and healthful breakfast attraction . . . or to help you survive a "snack attack" all by itself!

The complex carbohydrates featured in this power-packed recipe are utilized by the body at a steadier, more prolonged rate than are simple carbohydrates like sugar. The result is more prolonged energy for more sustained enjoyment of your chosen activities.

Here is how to make it:

¼ cup certified raw milk (or regular milk if you can't buy certified raw milk)

1 ripe banana

2 tablespoons raw, fresh wheat germ

2 tablespoons raw, hulled sunflower seeds

2 tablespoons nutritional yeast

3 of our famous oatmeal cookies (see recipe)

2 large scoops of natural, honey- or maple syrup-sweetened vanilla ice cream or ice milk (strawberry or carob ice cream is also good). Stores featuring health foods, whole foods, or gourmet foods usually carry ice creams like these.

Procedure:

Blend all ingredients in a blender for about 30 seconds. Drink slowly. (Don't forget the other goodies in this book make great companions for this dynamic drink.)

Variations: Our recipe does not call for any eggs, but you can add one if desired. A pint of vanilla yogurt can be substituted for the milk and ice cream.

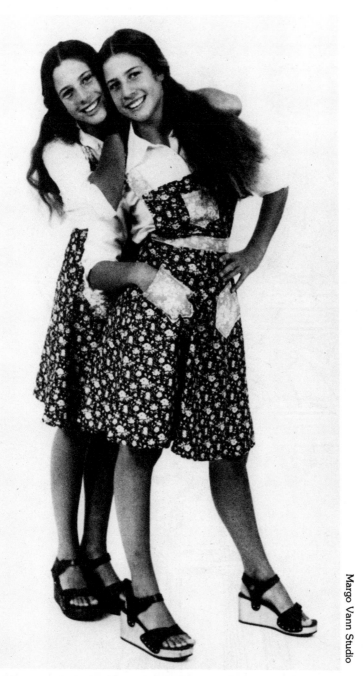

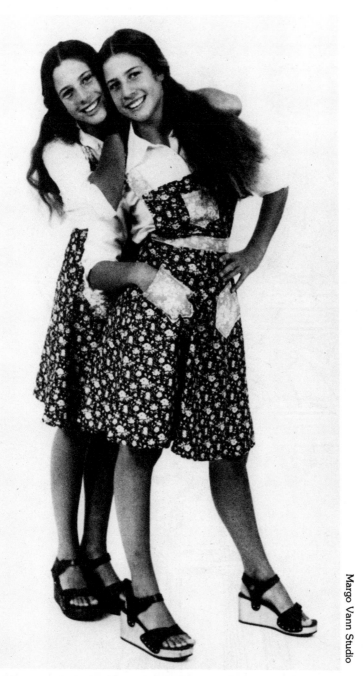

Margo Vann Studio

Double-energy, double fun . . . there is no substitute for the natural energy generated by your own healthy body made fit by good nutrition and avoiding harmful things.

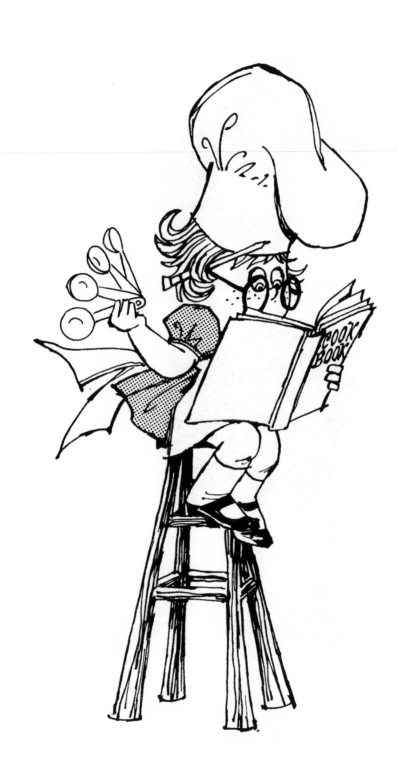

Recipes

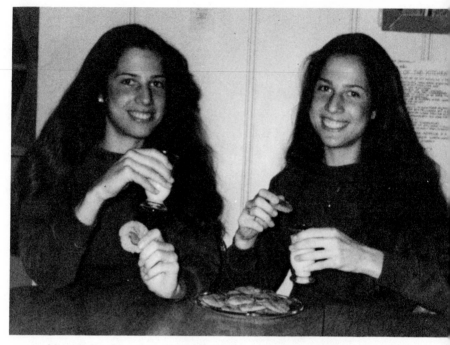

Having fun "surviving a snack attack . . . naturally," with a glass of milk
or our famous "double-your-energy" health drink as a super bonus.

Almond Cookies

¼ cup butter, softened
⅔ cup honey
2 teaspoons almond extract
1 teaspoon vanilla extract
1 egg
1½-1¾ cups whole wheat flour
    (or rice flour)
12 whole almonds

Procedure:

1. Mix all ingredients except almonds, adding flour last.

2. Drop in tablespoons on an oiled cookie sheet.

3. Split almonds in half, dip in honey and press into the center of cookies.

4. Bake at 300° F. for 10 minutes.

Makes about 23 cookies.

Baked Apples Stuffed with Nuts

4 cooking apples
1 cup chopped almonds
2 tablespoons melted butter
1 teaspoon cinnamon

Procedure:

1. Preheat oven to 375° F.

2. Core apples. Remove excess pulp from middle, while keeping outer skin and shape intact (keep pulp).

3. Mix almonds, melted butter and pulp. Spoon into apple cavities.

4. Place in ovenproof dish, sprinkle cinnamon on each apple and bake for about 30 minutes or until tender.

Toppings (if desired): Try whipping cream with honey or slice some cheese on top.

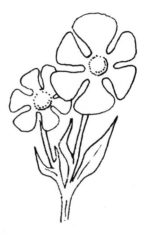

No-Cook Apple Cereal

2 cups old-fashioned rolled oats
½ cup raisins
3 apples, cored and cubed
3 cups applesauce
1½ cups milk

Procedure:

1. Mix all ingredients together.

Serves 4.

Apple-Banana Soynut Soother

2 red apples, cored and cubed
1 green apple, cored and cubed
2 ripe bananas, sliced
Plain yogurt
½ cup toasted soynuts

Procedure:

1. Mix fruit in salad bowl.

2. Add a few tablespoons of plain yogurt.

3. Sprinkle nuts on top.

Serves 4.

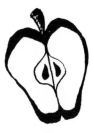

Apple Cookies

2 eggs
¼ cup whole wheat flour
¼ cup bran
¼ cup applesauce
1 teaspoon vanilla extract
3 apples, peeled, cored and chopped

Procedure:

1. Preheat oven to 350° F.

2. Place all the ingredients except the apples in a bowl and mix well.

3. Stir in apples.

4. Drop teaspoons of batter on an oiled baking sheet.

5. Bake about 15 minutes or until golden brown.

Yields about 2 dozen.

"Yummy" Apple Pie

Have double piecrust ready. Choose the crust that best suits your taste from our crust recipes on page 48.

Filling:

5 cups apples, cored and thinly sliced
2 tablespoons butter (optional)
2 tablespoons honey (optional)
¼ teaspoon cinnamon
½ teaspoon nutmeg
1 tablespoon wheat flour or wheat germ
½ cup chopped walnuts and/or raisins
      (optional)

Procedure:

1. Lay cored, thinly sliced apples on the crust.

2. Drizzle honey, then spices and flour over apples. (You can add walnuts and raisins if desired.) Put upper half of piecrust on top.

3. Bake at 350° F. for 45-60 minutes.

Variation: Spread applesauce on the bottom piecrust before putting in the filling.

Instant Applesauce

3 medium apples
1 tablespoon apple juice
½ teaspoon cinnamon
½ cup raisins (optional)

Procedure:

1. Core and dice apples. Puree in blender, a few pieces at a time.

2. As the apples are going through the blender, add apple juice.

3. Put freshly made applesauce in a bowl and sprinkle with cinnamon. Add raisins, if desired.

Serves 4.

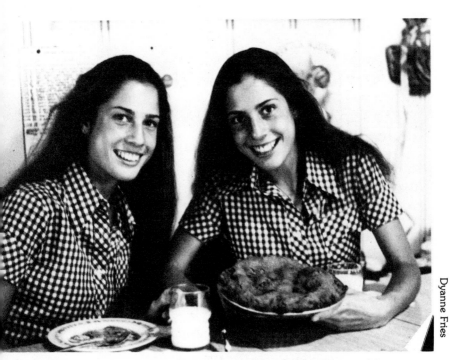

You'll be proud, too, when you bring a fantastic apple pie out of the oven—and know that a slice of it contains only natural goodness.

Apricot Bar Cookies

⅔ cup honey
½ cup oil
1 tablespoon lemon juice
1½ cups rolled oats
1 cup whole wheat flour
¾ cup wheat germ
1½ cups dried unsulfured apricots, chopped
½ cup sunflower seeds

Procedure:

1. Preheat oven to 350° F.

2. Beat together honey, oil and lemon juice.

3. In another bowl, combine oats, whole wheat flour and wheat germ.

4. Pour in honey mixture and mix until dry ingredients are moistened.

5. Add dried apricots and sunflower seeds.

6. Press into oiled 9-inch baking pan. Bake for 15-20 minutes. Cool in pan and cut into squares.

Banana-Coconut No-Bake Pie

Dash of nutmeg
2 cups sliced bananas
1¼ cups vanilla yogurt
½ cup toasted shredded coconut
1 large banana, sliced

Procedure:

1. Mix together nutmeg, bananas, and yogurt. Divide mixture into two parts.

2. Pour one-half of the mixture into a Coconut Sweet Piecrust (see "Crusts" on page 48).

3. Layer ½ large sliced banana and ¼ cup coconut over it. Then put in remaining mixture and cover again with remaining sliced bananas and coconut.

4. Put in refrigerator for 20 minutes.

Banana-Oatmeal Cookies

½ cup walnuts
⅓ cup honey
⅓ cup oil
1 egg
2 large bananas
1½ cups rolled oats
1¼ cups whole wheat flour
¼ teaspoon nutmeg
¾ teaspoon cinnamon

Procedure:

1. Grind nuts in a blender.

2. Separately blend honey, oil, egg and bananas. Combine with rest of ingredients to make a stiff batter.

3. Use a teaspoon to make cookies. Bake at 350° F. for about 15 minutes.

Makes 4 dozen cookies.

Berry Good Pie

3 cups chopped berries (preferably strawberries)
2 tablespoons strawberry preserves
1 egg, beaten
2 teaspoons wheat germ
½ teaspoon cinnamon
1 tablespoon oil
1 unbaked double piecrust

Procedure:

1. Preheat oven to 350° F.

2. Blend all ingredients.

3. Turn into unbaked piecrust.

4. Place upper part of pie crust on top of filling. Prick it in several places to allow steam to escape.

5. Bake for 30 minutes.

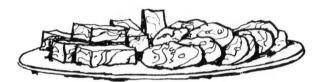

Brazil Nut Cookies

3 cups ground brazil nuts
2 eggs
¼ cup honey
½ teaspoon vanilla extract
¼ teaspoon kelp
2 tablespoons whole wheat pastry flour

Procedure:

1. Blend all ingredients. Chill for 2 hours.

2. Roll in small balls. Arrange on oiled cookie sheet.

3. Bake for 15 minutes at 325° F.

Butter Cookies

1 cup butter, softened
⅓ cup honey
2 yolks of hard-boiled eggs
1 raw egg yolk
3 cups whole wheat flour
1 tablespoon lemon juice

Procedure:

1. Blend all the ingredients together. (The dough will be a little stiff.)

2. Chill for an hour.

3. Roll out on floured board. Cut into round shapes and place on unoiled cookie sheet. Bake at 350° F. for about 10-12 minutes.

Yields 5 dozen cookies.

Carob Cookies

⅓ cup honey, slight
¼ cup plus 1 tablespoon oil
2 eggs, beaten
¼ cup whole wheat flour
5 tablespoons carob powder
1 teaspoon vanilla extract
2 tablespoons milk (optional)

Procedure:

1. Preheat oven to 350° F.

2. Blend honey, oil and eggs. Mix in flour, carob powder and vanilla. If moister cookie is desired, add 2 tablespoons milk.

3. Drop in teaspoonfuls onto lightly oiled cookie sheet. Bake for 10 minutes.

Yields 4 dozen small cookies.

Carob-Sunflower Cookies

Follow recipe for Carob Cookies. Add ¾ cup sunflower seeds (moistened and drained). Roll into balls, place on a lightly oiled cookie sheet, and press flat. Bake at 350° F. for about 12 minutes. This variation provides added texture and "chewiness."

Carob Cream Cheese Pie

¼ cup plus 2 tablespoons honey
2 3-ounce packages cream cheese, softened
4 eggs
1½ teaspoons vanilla extract
½ teaspoon lemon juice
5 tablespoons carob powder
1 cup chopped walnuts
1 single piecrust

Procedure:

1. Preheat oven to 350° F.

2. Blend together honey, cream cheese, eggs and vanilla. Add remaining ingredients.

3. Pour into piecrust. Bake for 40-45 minutes.

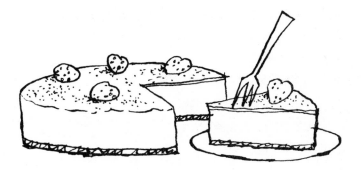

No-Bake Carob-Nut Drops

3 cups rolled oats
5 tablespoons carob powder
½ cup shredded coconut
½ cup chopped walnuts
1¼ cups honey
½ cup milk
½ cup butter

Procedure:

1. Combine oats, carob, coconut and nuts.

2. Put honey, milk and butter in a pan. Bring to a boil, stirring constantly.

3. Pour over rolled oats mixture. Mix lightly.

4. Drop in teaspoonfuls on waxed paper. Let stand until firm (about 10 minutes).

Yields about 4 dozen.

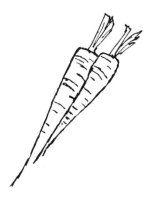

Carrot Pie

1 cup carrot juice
2 carrots, chopped
¼ cup wheat germ
¼ teaspoon cinnamon
⅓ cup raisins
½ cup chopped walnuts
1 double piecrust

Procedure:

1. Preheat oven to 350° F.

2. Mix all filling ingredients together.

3. Place in piecrust.

4. Put top half of crust on filling. Bake for 35 minutes.

Cashew-Coconut Cookies

¾ cup oil
⅔ cup honey
¾ cup milk
1¾ cups shredded coconut
1 cup raw chopped cashews
2 cups whole wheat flour
3 cups rolled oats
3 teaspoons vanilla extract

Procedure:

1. Preheat oven to 350° F.

2. Mix all ingredients in large bowl.

3. Drop in teaspoonfuls onto oiled baking sheet. Bake for about 10-12 minutes.

Makes about 5 dozen cookies.

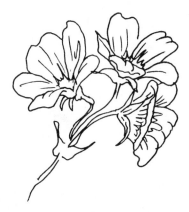

Coconut-Date Chews

3 eggs, well beaten
⅔ cup honey
1 cup pecans or walnuts
1 cup unsweetened shredded coconut
1 cup chopped dates
¾ cup whole wheat flour
¼ cup wheat germ
½ teaspoon lemon extract

Procedure:

1. Preheat oven to 350° F.

2. Combine all the ingredients and press down into a well-oiled 9-inch square baking pan.

3. Bake 15 minutes. Cut while warm.

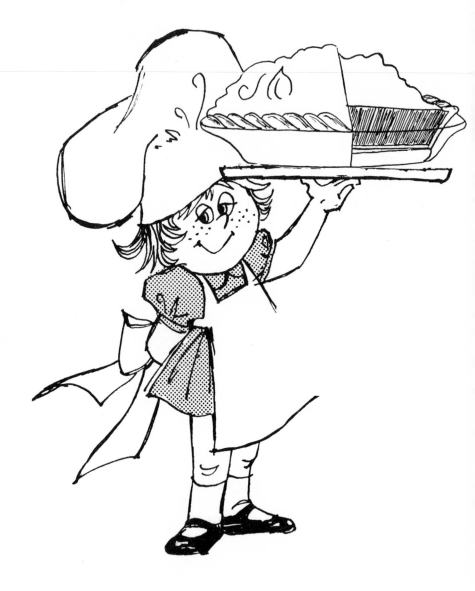

Crusts

Coconut Sweet Piecrust

1 cup raw wheat germ
¼ cup unsweetened coconut
¼ cup oil
1½ tablespoons honey
1 teaspoon cinnamon

Procedure:

1. Mix all ingredients together and press into 9-inch pie pan. This can be used raw or baked for 10 minutes at 325° F.

Cornmeal Crust

½ cup cornmeal
¾ cup whole wheat flour, sifted
½ teaspoon kelp
⅔ cup soft butter
4½ tablespoons cold water

Procedure:

1. Sift together cornmeal, flour and kelp.

2. Cut in butter until mixture resembles small peas.

3. Add water, 1 tablespoon at a time.

4. Roll out dough between 2 pieces of waxed paper or on a floured board.

5. Fit loosely into 9-inch pie plate.

6. Bake for 15 minutes at 350° F.

Rye Pie Shell

2 cups rye flour
½ teaspoon kelp
1 tablespoon chia seeds
½ cup oil
4 tablespoons ice water

Procedure:

1. Stir flour and kelp. Add seeds. Stir in oil.

2. Add ice water.

3. Press into 9-inch pie pan. Chill until ready to be filled and baked.

Whole Wheat Piecrust
(for top and bottom)

2 cups whole wheat flour, sifted
½ teaspoon kelp
⅔ softened butter or oil
¼ cup ice water
1 tablespoon lemon juice

Procedure:

1. Mix flour and kelp in a bowl.

2. Use fork or pastry blender to cut butter into flour until mixture is in pea-size chunks.

3. Mix ice water and lemon juice. Add liquid to dry ingredients, 1 tablespoon at a time.

4. Divide mixture in half and roll in between 2 pieces of waxed paper to about ⅛-inch thickness.

5. Bake crust for about 15 minutes at 400° F.

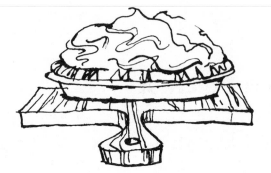

Whole Wheat-Rice Piecrust

¾ cup whole wheat flour
¾ cup rice flour
½ teaspoon kelp
½ cup oil
4 tablespoons cold water

Procedure:

1. Use same procedure as for making Whole Wheat Piecrust.

Cottage Cheese Filling

1 pint cottage cheese
3 tablespoons honey
2 eggs, separated
3 tablespoons lemon juice
¼ cup milk
1 single piecrust

Procedure:

1. Preheat oven to 350° F.

2. Blend cottage cheese with half the honey.

3. Add flour, egg yolks, lemon juice and milk.

4. Beat egg white stiff and add remaining honey.

5. Fold egg white mixture into cottage cheese.

6. Put in unbaked piecrust and bake for 35 minutes.

Cream Cheese Cookies

¼ cup honey
⅔ cup oil
½ cup cream cheese, softened
1 cup whole wheat flour
4 tablespoons sesame seeds
½ teaspoon lemon extract

Procedure:

1. Blend honey, oil and cream cheese.

2. Stir in flour and seeds. Add lemon extract.

3. Shape in long rolls and wrap in waxed paper. Chill for 2 hours.

4. Cut into thin slices. Bake for 5-10 minutes at 375° F.

Makes 2 dozen.

d

Date-Almond Cookies

2 eggs
1 cup butter
¼ cup honey
1 teaspoon almond extract
1½ cups chopped dates
1½ cups rolled oats
1½ cups whole wheat flour, sifted
½ teaspoon cinnamon
½ teaspoon nutmeg
⅔ cup milk
2 cups chopped almonds

Procedure:

1. Preheat oven to 350° F.

2. Beat eggs, butter, honey and almond extract together. Stir in dates and oats.

3. Sift together whole wheat flour, cinnamon and nutmeg. Gradually add milk. Stir in nuts.

4. Roll dough into small balls and press onto lightly oiled cookie sheet. Bake for 15 minutes.

Yield: More than 5 dozen cookies.

Date-Macaroon Cookies

1¼ cups shredded coconut
Little less than ½ cup honey
3 tablespoons oat flour
¼ cup chopped dates (or 3 store-bought ground-up dates rolled in coconut)
3 egg whites

Procedure:

1. Preheat oven to 300° F.

2. Mix everything but egg whites.

3. In a separate bowl beat egg whites until stiff.

4. Fold egg whites into the rest of the ingredients.

5. Drop by tablespoons onto an oiled cookie sheet. Bake for 10 minutes.

Yields 3 dozen.

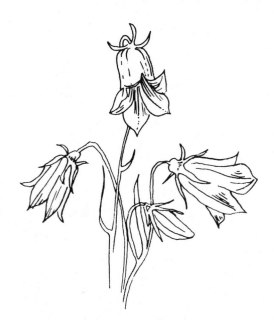

Date and Raisin Nut Balls

1 cup dates
2 tablespoons raisins
¼ cup chopped walnuts
1 tablespoon sunflower seeds
¼ cup powdered milk
Coconut

Procedure:

1. Run dried fruit through grinder with nuts. Mix in powdered milk.

2. Form into balls and roll in coconut.

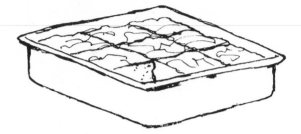

Date Squares

2 eggs, separated
2 tablespoons honey
1 teaspoon vanilla extract
½ cup flour
1 cup chopped walnuts
2 cups chopped dates

Procedure:

1. Preheat oven to 350° F.

2. Beat egg yolks, honey and vanilla. Mix in other ingredients.

3. Beat egg whites until stiff. Fold into mixture.

4. Bake in a small shallow pan for about 25 minutes. Cut into squares.

Dolly's Date-Nut Cookies

¾ cup butter, softened
2 eggs
1 cup honey
1 teaspoon vanilla extract
3 cups whole wheat flour, sifted
1 teaspoon kelp
4 tablespoons milk
2 cups pitted and cut dates
¾ cup chopped walnuts

Procedure:

1. Preheat oven to 350° F.

2. Blend butter, eggs, honey and vanilla.

3. Sift flour and kelp. Add to egg mixture.

4. Add milk while stirring mixture. Add dates and walnuts.

5. Drop in teaspoonfuls on oiled baking sheet. Cook for about 12 minutes.

Yields 5-6 dozen cookies.

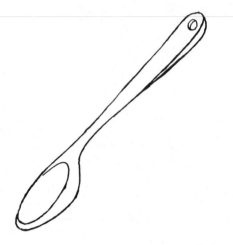

Eggless-Wheatless Oatmeal Cookies

3 cups rolled oats
⅓ cup soft butter (certified raw preferred)
¼ cup water
¼ cup honey
1 cup honey
1 teaspoon vanilla extract
1 teaspoon cinnamon

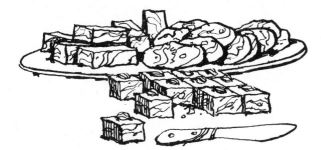

Procedure:

1. Preheat oven to 350° F.

2. Put 2 cups of the rolled oats in a blender and blend until it becomes "oat flour." Set aside.

3. With a spoon blend butter, water, honey and vanilla. Add the oat flour and the remaining cup of rolled oats. Sprinkle cinnamon over batter and mix.

4. Roll mixture into 1- or 1½-inch balls. Place on lightly oiled cookie sheet. Press flat. Bake for about 10 minutes. Makes 2 dozen cookies.

Variation: Add diced nuts or ½ cup sliced raisins or both.

Fig Cookies

2 cups finely chopped figs
1 cup oil
1 cup warm water
½ cup honey
1¾ cups whole wheat flour
½ cup wheat germ
1 cup chopped nuts
1 teaspoon vanilla extract

Procedure:

1. Preheat oven to 350° F.

2. Mix all ingredients together.

3. Drop by spoonfuls onto oiled cookie sheet. Bake for 10 minutes.

Yields about 2 dozen cookies.

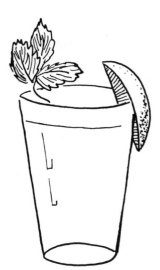

Fruit Coolies

Grape juice (or any fruit juice)
Ice trays

Procedure:

1. Pour juice in ice trays.

2. Place trays in freezer. Freeze.

3. Use little ice juice cubes to suck on or put them in your drinks!

4. Add sprig of fresh mint for aesthetic aroma and taste. Mint grows freely in a garden or even a window sill box.

Fudgy Carob

1 pound butter
2½ cups honey
2½ cups powdered milk
2 teaspoons vanilla extract
1½ cups carob powder

Procedure:

1. Melt butter, add honey and powdered milk until thick. Add vanilla.

2. Sift carob powder into creamy mixture and stir well. (This fudge is excellent with nuts and/or fruit.)

3. Put fudge in refrigerator to last longer.

g

Granola-Bran Cookies

¼ cup butter
½ cup honey
2 eggs, beaten
1 tablespoon lemon juice
1 cup whole wheat flour
½ cup bran
2 cups granola
1 cup chopped walnuts

Procedure:

1. Preheat oven to 375° F.

2. Cream together butter, honey, eggs and lemon juice.

3. Add flour, bran, granola and nuts.

4. Drop in teaspoonfuls onto oiled cookie sheet. Cook for about 8 minutes.

Yields about 3 dozen cookies.

Great Granola

½ cup honey
⅔ cup oil
2 pounds rolled oats
2 cups diced almonds
2 cups sunflower seeds
1 cup sesame seeds
½ cup chopped cashews
1 cup wheat germ

Procedure:

1. Preheat oven to 350° F.

2. Place honey and oil in a big cooking pot and heat.

3. Stir in dry ingredients and mix well.

4. Spread mixture over cookie sheets and cook for 12 minutes, stirring occasionally.

Makes PLENTY, so enjoy!

h

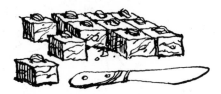

Halavah

3 cups hulled sesame seeds
1 cup hulled sunflower seeds, ground
Honey

Procedure:

1. Mix sunflower seeds and enough honey to hold mixture together.

2. Roll into sesame seeds. Form into little balls or bars and let sit out for an hour or so.
   Yummy candy!

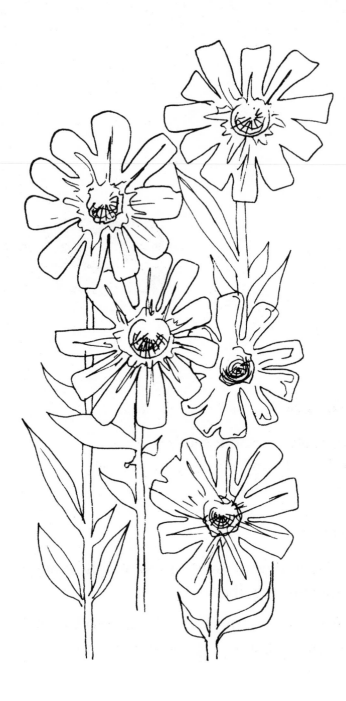

Lemon-Cashew Cookies

½ cup honey
¼ cup oil
3 tablespoons grated lemon rind
1 tablespoon lemon juice
2 eggs, beaten
1¾ cups whole wheat flour
½ cup wheat germ
2 teaspoons vanilla extract
¼ cup chopped raw cashews

Procedure:

1. Preheat oven to 350° F.

2. Blend honey and oil. Add lemon rind and lemon juice.

3. Add remaining ingredients except egg white and nuts.

4. Roll out stiff batter and cut into rounds. Sprinkle with cashews.

5. Place on cookie sheet. Bake about 10 minutes.

Yields 4 dozen cookies.

Lemon Meringue Pie

1 single piecrust, baked
3 tablespoons arrowroot
¼ cup and 1 tablespoon honey
⅛ teaspoon kelp
½ cup milk
½ cup cream
2 egg yolks (save whites for meringue)
1½ tablespoons butter
⅓ cup lemon juice
Grated rind of ½ lemon

Meringue

2 egg whites
½ teaspoon cream of tartar
½ teaspoon vanilla extract
1 teaspoon honey

Procedure:

1. Have pie crust precooked and ready to be filled.

2. In top of a double boiler, mix arrowroot, honey and kelp until smooth.

3. Have water boiling in bottom of double boiler. Reduce heat.

4. Slowly add milk and cream, stirring constantly, and continue cooking 8-10 minutes. Cover and let cook 10 minutes longer, stirring occasionally to keep from sticking.

5. In a separate bowl, beat egg yolks. Mix in a few tablespoons of hot mixture at a time. Then add yolks to mixture.

6. Remove from heat and add butter, lemon juice and lemon rind.

7. Stir gently, allowing steam to escape. Pour into empty pie crust.

Procedure for Meringue:

1. Preheat oven to 350° F.

2. Beat egg whites until nice stiff peaks appear.

3. Add cream of tartar vanilla and honey, and beat a little longer.

4. Cover filling with meringue and put pie in oven for about 10 minutes, until peaks turn to a golden brown.

Maple-Nut Meringue Cookies

2 egg whites
¼ cup maple syrup
½ teaspoon vanilla extract
¼ cup finely chopped walnuts
½ teaspoon cream of tartar
⅓ cup oat flour

Procedure:

1. Preheat oven to 275° F.

2. Beat egg whites until soft firm peaks are formed.

3. Add maple syrup, continue to beat, and fold in vanilla, walnuts and tartar. Add flour.

4. Cover a baking sheet with foil. Drop meringue in tablespoonfuls with little peaks.

5. Place in oven, reducing heat to 250° F., and bake for 30 minutes.

6. Let cookies cool and peel off paper foil.

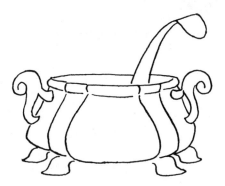

Melon Mama Supreme

1 cup cubed watermelon
½ cup cubed cantaloupe
½ cup cubed honeydew melon
1 cup whipping cream
Honey
½ cup chopped nuts

Procedure:

1. Place cubed melons in a bowl and set aside.

2. In another bowl whip whipping cream and add just enough honey for sweetener.

3. Pour whipped cream on fruit. Sprinkle with nuts. Chill.

Serves 4.

Oatmeal Cookies

⅔ cup soft butter
1 cut honey
1 egg
¼ cup water
1 teaspoon vanilla extract
1 cup whole wheat flour
3 cups rolled oats
½ teaspoon cinnamon

Procedure:

1. Preheat oven to 350° F.

2. Beat butter, honey, egg, water and vanilla together until somewhat creamy.

3. Add remaining ingredients. Mix well.

4. Drop by teaspoonfuls onto oiled cookie sheet. Bake for about 12 minutes.

Variation: For eggless oatmeal cookies, just eliminate the egg.

Yields about 5 dozen cookies.

p

Peanut Butter Cookies

¼ cup oil
½ cup honey
1¼ cups whole wheat flour
½ cup peanut butter
¼ cup wheat germ
1 teaspoon vanilla extract

Procedure:

1. Preheat oven to 350° F.

2. Mix all ingredients. Drop from a teaspoon onto cookie sheet and flatten with a fork.

3. Bake about 10 minutes.

Yields about 20 cookies.

Peanut Butter Treats
(uncooked)

½ cup peanut butter
2 tablespoons nutritional yeast
¾ cup wheat germ
¼ cup golden raisins (unsulfured)
¾ cup puffed wheat

Procedure:

1. Mix peanut butter, yeast, wheat germ and raisins together.

2. Roll into balls with puffed wheat.

3. Eat the treats right away, or chill them.

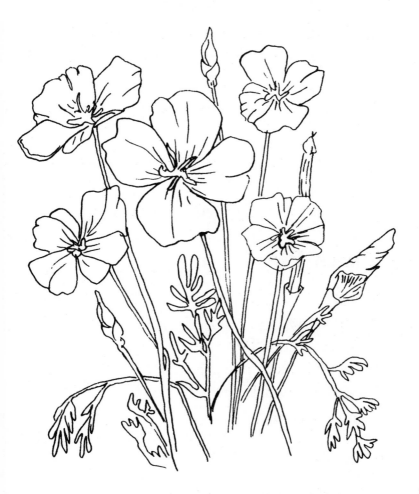

Pecan Pie

3 eggs
⅔ cup honey
¼ cup butter, softened
1½ cups broken pecans
1 teaspoon vanilla extract
1 single piecrust

Procedure:

1. Preheat oven to 375° F.

2. Mix eggs, honey and butter.

3. Add pecans and vanilla and mix well.

4. Bake in pie shell for 20-25 minutes.

This pie is quite tasty with fresh whipped cream or vanilla yogurt.

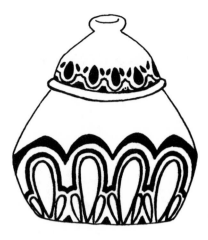

Pretty Pistachios

¼ cup and 1 tablespoon oil
2 eggs, beaten
¼ cup honey
¼ cup milk
¾ cup ground pistachios
1 cup whole wheat flour
1 cup oat flour

Procedure:

1. Preheat oven to 350° F.

2. Blend oil, eggs and honey.

3. Add milk, nuts and flours.

4. Drop by teaspoonfuls onto cookie sheet.
Bake for about 14 minutes.

Yields about 2 dozen cookies.

Popcorn

¾ cup popping corn kernels
¼ cup oil

Procedure:

1. Get a heavy pot with a good lid. Place oil and kernels in it.

2. Turn on medium/high heat.

3. After you hear the first kernel pop, let it keep popping for about 5 minutes.

Popcorn tastes great with: melted butter, melted butter and honey, peanut butter, peanuts and raisins, dried fruit, and in salads or sandwiches!

Pumpkin Cookies

¼ cup butter
¾ cup honey
2 eggs
1 cup mashed, steamed pumpkin pulp
 (canned or fresh)
1¾ cups whole wheat flour
¼ cup wheat germ
2 teaspoons cinnamon
1¾ cups chopped pecans

Procedure:

1. Preheat oven to 350° F.

2. Cream butter, honey, eggs and pumpkin together.

3. Mix in dry ingredients and nuts.

4. Drop by teaspoonfuls onto oiled cookie sheet. Bake for 12 minutes.

Yields a little more than 2 dozen cookies.

Pumpkin Pie

1 cup steamed pumpkin pulp (canned or fresh)
½ cup milk
2 eggs
¼ cup honey
¼ cup powdered milk
¼ teaspoon ginger
¼ teaspoon cinnamon
⅛ teaspoon nutmeg
1 teaspoon vanilla extract
1 single piecrust

Procedure:

1. Preheat oven to 350° F.

2. Combine all ingredients. Mix until smooth and pour into piecrust. Bake for about 40 minutes, until the filling is firm.

Raisin 'n' Spice Cookies

2 eggs, well beaten
1 cup honey
1 tablespoon milk
1 teaspoon cinnamon
¼ teaspoon cloves
½ teaspoon nutmeg
¾ cup butter, softened
2¼ cups whole wheat flour, sifted
1 cup raisins, cut in pieces
½ cup chopped nuts

Procedure:

1. Preheat oven to 350°F.

2. Beat eggs, honey and milk together.

3. Combine spices and butter. Blend into egg mixture.

4. Add sifted flour. Then mix in raisins and nuts.

5. Drop in teaspoonfuls onto cookie sheet. Bake for about 12 minutes.

Yields 5 dozen cookies.

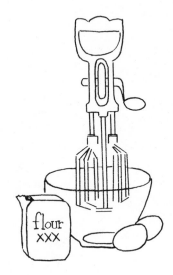

Sesame Cookies

2 eggs
½ cup honey
2 tablespoons oil
1½ cups whole wheat flour
1 tablespoon lecithin
½ cup sesame seeds
1 teaspoon vanilla extract

Procedure:

1. Preheat oven to 350° F.

2. Beat eggs, add honey and oil. Mix well.

3. Add flour, lecithin and sesame seeds. Add vanilla.

4. Drop by teaspoonfuls onto oiled cookie sheet. Cook for about 14 minutes.

Yields 30 cookies.

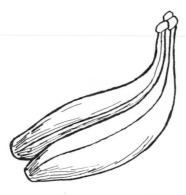

Sour Cream Banana Rolls

½ cup sour cream
2 ripe bananas, sliced
¼ cup shredded coconut
Toothpicks

Procedure:

1. Dip sliced bananas in sour cream.

2. Roll bananas in shredded coconut.

3. Place a toothpick in each slice of banana and put them on a tray. Chill.

Serves 4

Shari's Soy Cookies

¼ cup butter
1 tablespoon vanilla extract
⅔ cup honey
2 eggs
3 tablespoons soy flour
1 cup roasted soybeans, ground
½ cup roasted soybeans, chopped
2 tablespoons wheat germ (optional)

Procedure:

1. Preheat oven to 300° F.

2. Blend butter, vanilla and honey.

3. Blend in eggs. Stir in flour and soybeans. Add wheat germ if desired.

4. Drop in teaspoonfuls onto oiled cookie sheet. Bake for 10 minutes.

Yields a dozen cookies.

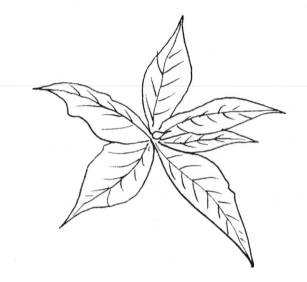

Soynut Cheese Balls

1 3-ounce package cream cheese, softened
3 tablespoons crushed pineapple, drained
¼ teaspoon kelp
¼ cup toasted soynuts, finely chopped

Procedure:

1. Mix cream cheese, pineapple and kelp.

2. Form into balls and roll into soynuts.

3. Chill.

Makes about 8 servings.

Sunny Macaroons

1¼ cups honey
1 cup sunflower seeds, hulled
3½ cups shredded coconut
½ cup whole wheat flour
¼ cup chopped dried apple
6 egg whites, beaten stiff

Procedure:

1. Preheat oven to 300° F.

2. Blend honey, sunflower seeds, shredded coconut, flour and apple.

3. Fold in egg whites.

4. Drop by teaspoonfuls onto oiled cookie sheet. Bake for about 25 minutes.

Yields 4 dozen.

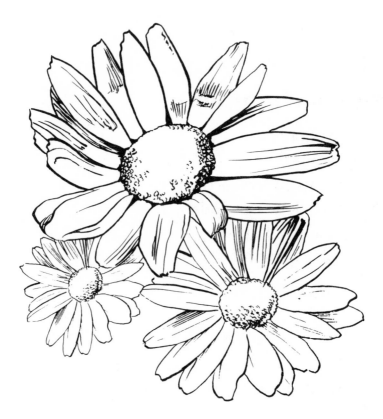

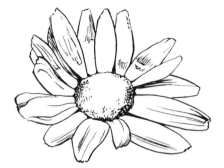

Vanilla Filbert Cookies

⅓ cup safflower oil
¼ cup honey
1 egg beaten
1 tablespoon vanilla
¾ cup sifted whole wheat flour
24 filberts

Procedure:

1. Blend oil, honey, egg and vanilla. Stir in flour.

2. Roll into small balls and press each cookie down while placing a filbert in the middle.

3. Bake at 350° F. on an oiled cookie sheet for 10-12 minutes.

Yields 24 cookies.

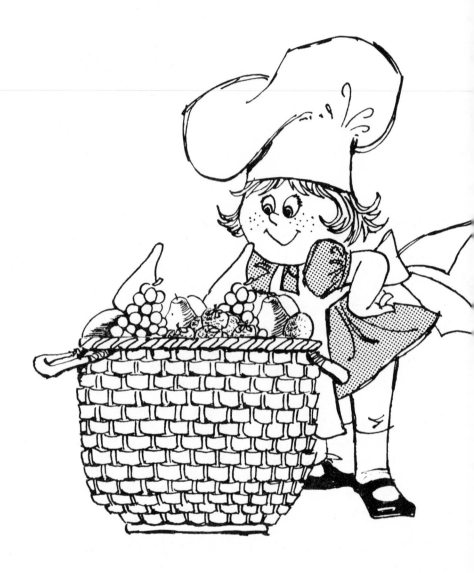

Yogurt Cookies

¼ cup honey
2 tablespoons oil
1 teaspoon vanilla extract
2 eggs
⅓ cup plain yogurt
1 cup whole wheat flour
¼ cup wheat germ
2 tablespoons bran
½ cup currants (or raisins)

Procedure:

1. Preheat oven to 350° F.

2. Blend honey, oil, vanilla, eggs and half the yogurt.

3. When well blended, stir in rest of the yogurt and flour, wheat germ and bran. Mix in currants.

4. Drop by teaspoonfuls onto oiled cookie sheet. Bake for about 8-10 minutes.

Yields 2 dozen cookies.

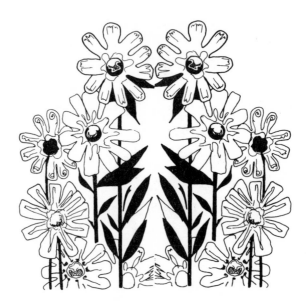

Helpful Hints

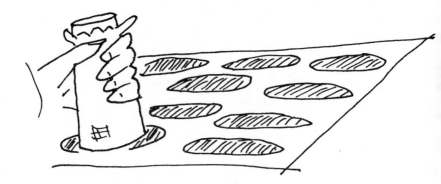

Helpful Hints for Cookies

1. Pressing the dough down with a damp cloth wrapped around the bottom of a glass will make perfect shaped cookies.

2. When using eggs, we suggest that you beat them well to increase the fluffiness of the cookie, since we don't use baking powder or soda.

3. If you use granular lecithin in cookies, reduce the amount of oil a little.

4. Always check your cookies. Don't just leave them baking for the required time. Make sure they aren't burning.

5. Important: always check cookies halfway through their baking time and turn them over. An undercooked cookie is better than an overcooked one.

6. To test if cookies are done, touch them lightly. If no fingerprint remains, they are ready.

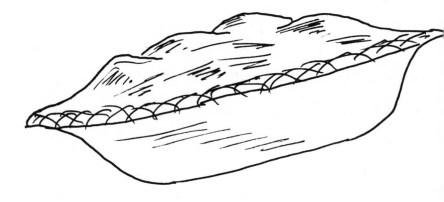

Helpful Hints for Pies

1. To vary the flavor of the piecrusts, one can reduce the amount of whole wheat flour by a couple of tablespoons and substitute soy, rye, oat, or even rice flour.

2. Sometimes an egg added to the dough keeps the piecrust together and more consistent.

3. Piecrusts are usually easier to handle if they are chilled before rolling them between wax paper or on a pastry cloth.

4. When putting a top on your pies, always cut a couple of slits on the top to allow steam to escape.

5. When the pie is baking for more than 20 minutes, we suggest you wrap some aluminum foil around the crust so that it doesn't burn.

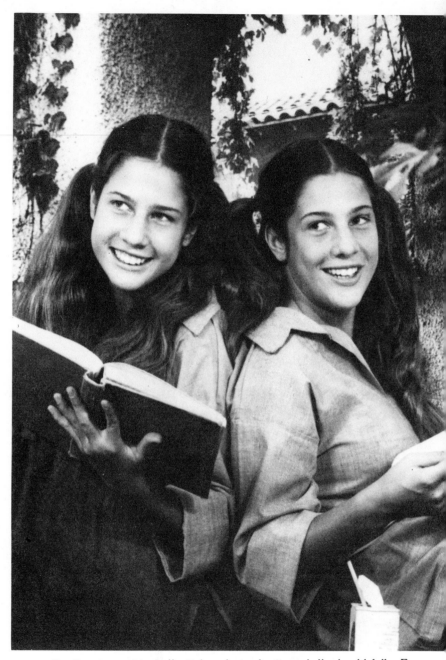

Our "neat sweet treats" satisfy a desire for "snacks"—healthfully. For lasting vitality you also need a well-balanced, natural diet. When you really study the basics of good nutrition, you'll agree that Dr. Paavo Airola's Optimum Diet is just that—the best.

We Salute

Dr. Paavo Airola's Optimum Diet

These nutritious cookies and pies are part of our diet, but we always make sure we eat completely balanced nutritious meals. Our diet is primarily based on the "Airola Optimum Diet" by Paavo Airola, N.D., Ph.D.

Dr. Airola, the world-famous nutritionist, has seven basic rules for his "Optimum Diet," which we would like to pass on to our readers because we have great respect for Dr. Airola and his teachings:

(1) Eat Only Natural Foods

Try to get foods grown on fertile soil under natural conditions, instead of chemically treated foods. Avoid synthetic, denatured, altered and devitalized foods.

(2) Eat Only Whole Foods

Whole foods contain all the nutrients nature has put into them, no more and no less. Avoid white bread, instant potatoes, polished rice and white sugar. Whole foods not only contain complete nutrition and vitamins, but also all the enzymes and other factors necessary for proper, effective digestion and good assimilation of each particular food.

(3) Eat Only Living Foods

Cooking totally destroys enzymes. Enzymes are essential for proper digestion and assimilation of food as well as for all functions in one's body. Minerals are also lost in cooking food. Water-soluble vitamins B and C are particularly vulnerable to the effect of heat and cooking. Nuts and seeds should be eaten raw for better digestion, but grains can be cooked, as in breads and cereals. Sprouts are .excellent, too. At least two-thirds of all foods should be eaten raw. If cooking is absolutely necessary, food should be cooked as little as possible.

(4) Eat Only Poison-Free Foods

Fruits and vegetables contain residues of dozens of poisonous pesticides, waxes, bleaches, preservatives and other artificial ingredients. Meat, milk, butter and poultry contain, in addition to DDT and other insecticides, residues of hormones, antibiotics and other drugs used to increase animal growth. Processed foods are loaded with thousands of different chemicals. Every effort, therefore, should be made to obtain poison-free organically grown foods. Most health food stores and some supermarkets provide quality produce. The produce should be washed carefully in either soap or salt water or in a 3% solution of hydrochloric acid and then brushed clean with a vegetable brush.

(5) Eat High Natural Carbohydrate-Low Animal Protein Diet

The most perfectly balanced diet is a diet rich in organically grown fruits and vegetables and raw or sprouted whole grains, seeds or nuts. Lactovegetarians can use certified raw unpasteurized milk, yogurt and homemade cottage cheese from organically fed animals. Fortified with cold-pressed vegetable oils, honey, wheat germ and bran, brewer's yeast, kelp and dry fruits, this high natural carbohydrate-low animal protein diet will supply one with all the required nutrients: vitamins, minerals, trace elements, enzymes, proteins, fatty acids, carbohydrates and other vital substances in a natural, pure and easily assimilated form.

(6) Systematic Undereating and Periodic Fasting

Poor digestion and assimilation of nutrients caused by overeating causes nutritional deficiencies. Moderation is the key word in order for food to be efficiently digested and better utilized. "Moderation" is a key word for eating as well as doing anything in life!

(7) Correct Eating Habits

Food should be eaten slowly. It is far better to skip a meal than to eat in a hurry. Well-chewed and generously salivated food is practically half-digested before it enters the stomach. Eat in a relaxed atmosphere, also.

As far as food mixing is concerned, the entire food-mixing "science" of this "Airola Optimum Diet" can be summed up in a few lines:

1. Never eat raw fruits and raw vegetables at the same meal.
2. Eat as few different foods as possible at one meal.
3. When protein-rich foods are eaten with other foods, eat the protein foods first.

We believe in what Dr. Paavo Airola has to say about proper nutrition. Everybody's metabolism is somewhat different, but we feel by following the "Airola Optimum Diet" one will feel better and appreciate life much more.

If you're interested in reading more about Dr. Airola's nutritional writings, we highly recommend *How to Get Well, Hypoglycemia: A Better Approach* and *Are You Confused?* These books can be found in most health food stores or can be ordered from the publishers of this book or directly from Health Plus Publishers, P. O. Box 22001, Phoenix, Arizona 85028. Dr. Airola has also written ten other best-selling books.

When the Dessert "Deserts" . . .

The Exercise Begins!

Now that you've read our healthy "Snack Attacks" cookbook, don't just think you can lie back and stuff yourself. You have to work some of those calories off.

We aren't telling you to do all the exercise that we do, but it would be helpful and healthful if you added some exercise to your daily regime.

Besides basic stretches, it's an excellent idea to take a brisk walk for a half-hour or so, or swim a few laps, or just go on a bike ride to do some errands.

We try to run anywhere from two to five miles a day, plus ride our bike (ours is built for two!) all over the place. We also love to swim. Daily exercise not only helps one's looks, but it seems to help one's total mental attitude.

A good idea for one who is not used to exercising a lot would be to start off on an easy exercise program and gradually build up. Don't be an *H.M.W.* (Haste Makes Waster), one who starts off running six miles a day and expects fast results. The only fast results one may receive from being an H.M.W. may be a lot of pain. Remember, the best things in life are those that require time and effort.

A balanced diet of wholesome foods and daily exercise will contribute to a long and satisfying Life. Don't wait until it's too late. The best time is NOW!

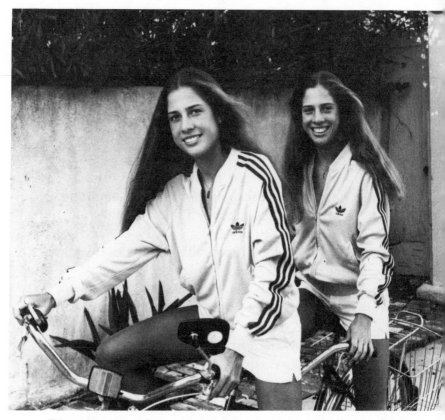

Bike riding is good exercise for almost everyone. We do it in double time on our bicycle built for two.

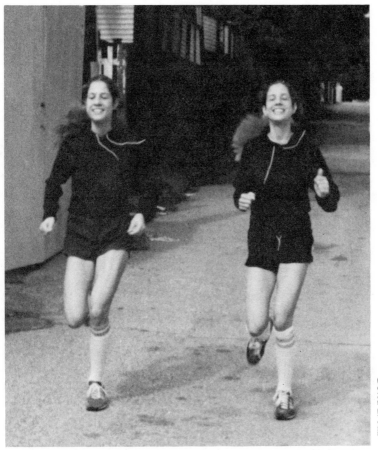

Devra Z. Hill

One of the best exercises of all—and one of the most popular is just running. If you are a little older than we are or if you have a health problem, you'll want to check with your doctor first, but for most people, running is almost the perfect exercise—and good, brisk walking is almost as good.

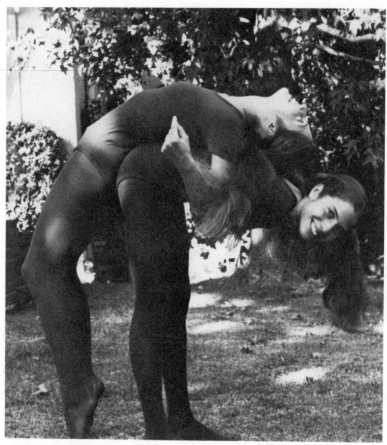

Depending on your age and condition, old-fashioned gymnastics or just "setting up" exercises provide a good, quick workout.

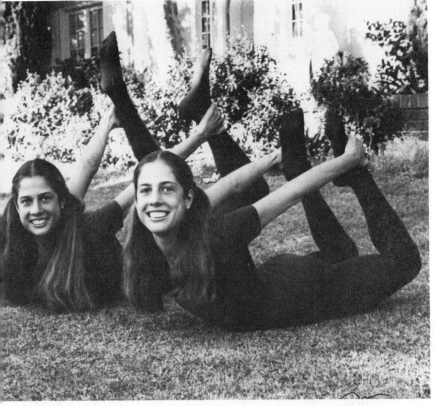

Dyanne Fries

We are each fortunate to have a "close partner" that makes exercising more fun for us. But some people prefer to exercise alone. Either way, it will make you more fit—and more fun!

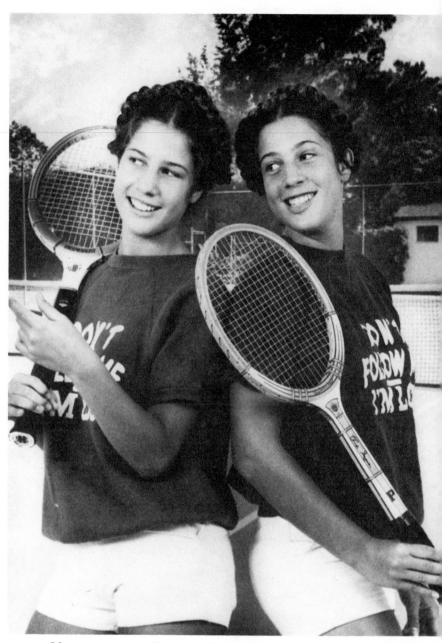

Most active sports, like tennis, have a lot of exercise value—probably not as complete as running or swimming but the enjoyment of the sport may lead you to exercise more—and that's a plus.

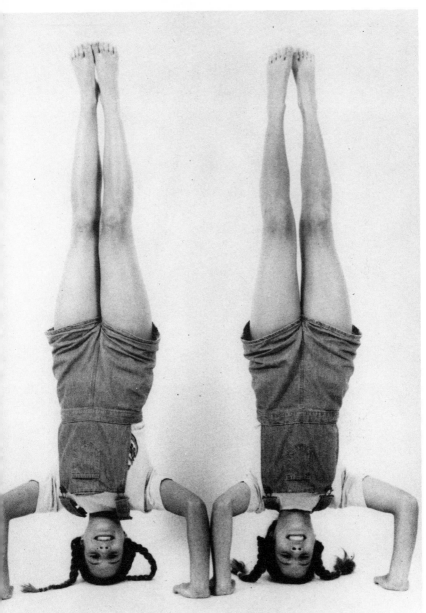

You may not want to try this, but in some manner or other you have to keep your body active in order to be healthy.

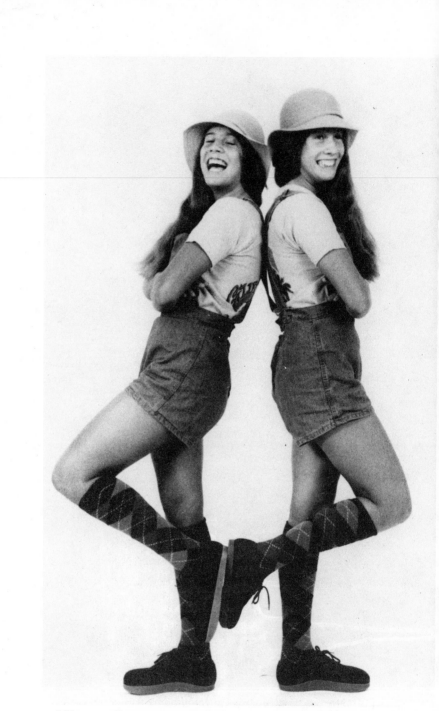

Hiking, walking, running, biking, gymnastics—anything that helps to keep you active will help you have a more invigorated body, a keener mind, and a healthier and longer life!